THE
LOW RESIDUE DIET
COOKBOOK

-----------------~----------------

70 Low Residue (Low Fiber) Healthy Homemade Recipes for People with IBD, Diverticulitis, Crohn's Disease & Ulcerative Colitis

-----------------~----------------

ALSO INCLUDES: DETAILED NUTRITIONAL INFORMATION FOR EACH RECIPE

BY

MONIKA SHAH

COPYRIGHT © 2015

A Message for Readers!

Low Residue Diet for Diverticulitis, IBD, Crohn's disease & Ulcerative colitis

This book has been specifically designed and written for people who have been suffering with bowel inflammation or diagnosed with inflammatory bowel disease, also known as IBD, Crohn's disease (a chronic inflammatory disease of the intestines), Ulcerative colitis or Diverticulitis and advised to follow a **Low Residue Diet** (Low Fiber Diet). It is extremely important to eat the right food types and diet during this course to ease the discomfort caused.

Let's take a closer look on what this book has to offer:

- **The Low Residue Diet Cookbook:** The cookbook has 70 Low residue (Low Fiber) and healthy homemade recipes which are designed especially for people who have been suffering with IBD, Crohn's disease, Ulcerative colitis or Diverticulitis.

  The recipes in the book have been designed using very simple ingredients that people use in their kitchen every day or can find in the grocery stores very easily. These recipes are further categorized into **Main Dishes, Sides Dishes, Beverages and Desserts.**

- **Healthy & Delicious Recipes:** The whole purpose of these recipes is to make sure that the person suffering with either IBD, Crohn's disease, Ulcerative colitis or Diverticulitis enjoys life without compromising the taste of the real food.

  Each recipe in this book has easy to find ingredients and steps with accurate serving sizes and detailed nutritional values. You will find recipes which can be eaten daily or on occasions without even compromising with health a bit.

- **Accurate Nutritional Information:** Each recipe comes with an accurate Nutritional Information Table to help people know what nutrition (especially Fiber) they are getting and in what quantities. The nutritional table of each recipe provides "Amounts per serving" details for:

  - *Calories*
  - *Trans Fat*
  - *Sodium*
  - *Protein*
  - *Cholesterol*
  - *Potassium*
  - *Total Fat*
  - *Carbohydrates*
  - *Phosphorus*
  - *Saturated Fat*
  - *Fiber*
  - *Calcium.*

CONTENTS

Copyright Notes & Disclaimer

This Page Has Been Left Blank Intentionally.

Chapter 1

Understanding Low Residue Diet (Low Fiber Diet)

The term "**Residue**" refers to the indigestible content of food we eat. Foods that contain a residue increase the stool weight and the fecal residue. Such foods are therefore to be avoided if you need to be on a low residue diet. Foods that are high in residue include high fiber foods like fruits and vegetables. You may also need to avoid tough and fibrous meats with gristle (an animal tissue that is difficult to digest) as they add to more residues and hence must be avoided.

A low residue diet contains foods that are very easy to digest, pass and do not cause a blockage. On a low residue diet it is important to avoid foods that are high in fiber content. The term "**Fiber**" refers to the portion of carbohydrates (starch) that humans cannot digest. Fiber passes through the digestive tract mostly unchanged and hence not recommended during low residue diet.

Generally, foods that contain fiber content help the movement of fluid and food through the gut. These foods also add bulk to the stool and are usually recommended as part of a healthy diet. However, it is advisable to avoid these foods in certain conditions and/or in preparation for particular procedures because they can leave behind a 'residue' after digestion.

You may also need to follow a low residue diet for one of the following reasons:

- **Narrowing of the gut**: You may have developed a narrowing of the gut, also known as Stricture. Stricture means that foods containing fiber may not pass through your gut easily and may cause a blockage. In such a condition, a low residue diet is recommended to avoid bulky stools.

- **Gut lining wall inflammation**: A disease or radiotherapy has caused an inflammation of the lining of the gut wall. In this condition, foods containing high fiber content may aggravate the gut and lead to diarrhea.

- **Medical investigation or procedure**: You may be asked to follow a low residue diet if you have some kind of bowel inflammation and a medical investigation or procedure must be carried out to investigate.

- **Reintroduction of food**: A low residue diet may also be recommended by doctors and dieticians after a surgery. In some cases, you may also be asked to follow a low residue diet after completing a course of liquid diet program.

Other conditions where a low residue diet may be recommended are **Crohn's disease (a chronic inflammatory disease of the intestines), Ulcerative colitis, Bowel inflammation** and **Diverticulitis**.

Some people think that these conditions are caused due to high fiber food which is not the case. A high fiber diet should always be followed by a human being, as it adds to a better health. But if you are suffering from any of the diseases mentioned above, avoiding high fiber foods may make you feel more comfortable.

In other words, if you need to follow a low residue diet, you must reduce the amount of fiber you eat. Low fiber intake leads to low residue and helps in healing the bowel inflammation comfortably without pain.

Basic Principles of a Low Residue Diet

There are some basic principles of low residue diet that one should always follow. These are in addition to the foods that should not be consumed during the course of a low residue diet. Let's take a quick look at these principles:

- A low fiber diet must not contain more than 10-15 grams of fiber per day.
- Foods with some fiber like fruits and vegetable must be well cooked.
- Avoid highly seasoned foods. It is not required to completely stop seasoning the food. You just need to make sure that the food is seasoned in moderation.
- Avoid eating large meals as they may cause discomfort from gastric distention.
- Avoid frying completely and try to cook by baking, boiling, broiling, roasting, stewing, microwaving, or creaming.

As far as the length of low residue diet is concerned, it is used temporarily until your digestive processes normalize. Once normalized, you can resume with your regular diet, only avoiding foods that you cannot normally tolerate.

This Page Has Been Left Blank Intentionally.

Chapter 2

Guidelines to Control Your Fiber Intake

During the course of a low residue diet, people need to be smart and follow certain guidelines. These guidelines are provided to help people choose foods that are low in fiber content and do not leave residue. Use these guidelines as high level principles while following a low residue diet. *Please refer to chapter 3 for a detailed list of foods that should be included and avoided in the diet.*

Let's take a look at these guidelines.

- Buy and use white cereals such as rice based cereals and cornflakes.
- Buy and use cereal products prepared without seeds and nuts.
- Buy and use white or refined bread without nuts, seeds and grains.
- Buy and use white varieties of pasta and rice.
- Buy and use plain white biscuits such as malted milks, rich tea and custard creams.
- Buy and use white varieties scones and crumpets.
- You must always cook the vegetables well from the allowed foods list. Please refer to Chapter 3 for the list of allowed vegetables.
- You can use herbs and spices that are ground finely.
- People who have ostomy must avoid highly seasoned food and especially garlic cloves. Garlic powder can be consumed in moderation.
- Remove the skin of potatoes before using.

- If you bake at home, always use white flour.
- Try not to consume vegetables and fruits with skins, pips and seeds as they are high in fiber and leaves residue.
- You may try to boil and puree fruits and vegetables. If they don't suit you, stop eating them.
- Always make sure the soups, sauces and meals that you buy from the stores do not have added fruits, vegetables, seeds and nuts in them.
- During the course of low residue diet, you will be restricting a lot of fruits and vegetables which may lead to vitamin C deficiency. Make sure you include and drink a vitamin C rich fresh fruit juice (without bits) or squash every day.
- Do not eat more than 3 servings of fruits per day from the allowed list of fruits provided in chapter 3.
- Always use ground, well cooked or tender poultry, fish, lamb, pork, ham, veal, beef and eggs.
- Do not eat fried and tough, fibrous meats with gristle.
- Avoid highly seasoned sausages and cold cut meats, also known as luncheon meats.
- You may consume tea, coffee and fruit punch in moderation.
- It is recommended that a standard multivitamin with minerals is taken daily. You can check with your doctor or certified dietician on this.
- You can eat deserts and sweets without fruits and nuts. Please refer to chapter 3 for a detailed list of allowed sweets and deserts.

Avoiding these foods will aid in pain free bowel movement and inflammation. It is important that one should know about each and every food and food type that adds to more residues. Please read through chapter 3 to find more about foods and food groups that should be included and avoided during a low residue diet program.

Chapter 3

Foods to Include & Exclude in Low Residue Diet

Unlike other diet programs, low residue diet offers a wide variety of foods that can be consumed. In this chapter you will be able to identify the list of foods from various food groups that should be included to and avoided from a low residue diet program. Let's have a look at these foods and food groups in detail.

Breads and Starches

The following is a list of allowed and not allowed foods for Breads and Starches food group.

Allowed Foods	Foods to Avoid
- White breads	- Wholemeal bread and flour
- Muffins	- Granary bread and flour
- Rolls	- Wholemeal pasta
- Biscuits	- Quinoa
- Crackers	- Pearl barley
- Light rye bread (seedless)	- Brown rice
- Pancakes	- All cereals that contain whole wheat
- Waffles	- Muesli
- Corn flakes	- Porridge
- Special k	- All foods that contain nuts

	and dried fruits
- Rice krispies	
- Puffed rice	
- White potatoes	
- Sweet potatoes (without skin)	
- White rice	
- Pasta	
Refined cooked cereals like:	
- Cream of rice	
- Cream of wheat	
- Farina	
- Grits	

Note: Products that are made with coconut, nuts, bran, seeds or dried fruits are very high in fiber and leave a great amount of residue and hence not recommended in this diet.

Meat and Protein

The following is a list of allowed and not allowed foods for Meat and Protein food group.

Allowed Foods	Foods to Avoid
- Ground, tender or well cooked meats	- Tough and gristly meat
- Poultry	- Skin and bones of fish
- Tofu	- Pies containing vegetables
- Fish	- Egg dishes containing vegetables (as listed in the allowed vegetables section, later in this chapter)

- Eggs	
- Creamy peanut butter	**Legumes (peas and beans)**
	- Kidney beans
	- Lima beans
	- Navy beans
	- Black beans
	- Soy beans
	- Split black eyed beans
	- Chickpeas
	- Garbanzo
	- Pinto beans
	- Peanuts
	- Yellow peas
	- Lentils
	- Crunchy peanut butter

Vegetables

The following is a list of allowed and not allowed foods for Vegetables food group.

Allowed Foods	Foods to Avoid
- Cucumber	- Raw vegetables and salads
- Green pepper	- Split peas
- Romaine	- Lentils
- Tomatoes	- Peas
- Onions	- Sweet corn
- Zucchini	- Celery
	- All seeds
	- All pips
	- All tough skins
	- Potato skins

	- Baked beans
	- Lima beans
	- Green peas
	- Broccoli
	- Parsnips
	- All others
	- Juices with pulp or bits

Note: All vegetables are allowed except the ones that are not recommended.

Fruits

The following is a list of allowed and not allowed foods for Fruits food group.

Allowed Foods	Foods to Avoid
- Apricot	- All dried fruits
- Peach	- Citrus fruit
- Plum	
- Honeydew	**Berries**
- Nectarine	- Strawberries
- Papaya	- Blackberries
- Banana	- Raspberries
- Cantaloupe	
- Watermelon	- Prunes
- All juices without pulp and strained	- All Smoothies
	- Fruit juices with bits

Note: All fruits are allowed except the ones that are not recommended or those with seeds or skins.

Dairy Products

The following is a list of allowed and not allowed foods for Dairy food group.

Allowed Foods	Foods to Avoid
- Yogurt	- Products with seeds and nuts in them
- Cheese	
- Milk	

Fats

The following is a list of allowed and not allowed foods for Fats food group.

Allowed Foods	Foods to Avoid
- Butter	- Nuts
- Bacon	- Seeds
- Salad dressings	- Coconut
- Vegetable oils	- Olives
- Mayonnaise	- Poppy seed dressings
- Margarine	- Crunchy peanut butter
- Cream	
- Whip cream	
- Plain gravies	
- Creamy peanut butter	

Sweets & Deserts

The following is a list of allowed and not allowed foods for Sweets and Deserts food group.

Allowed Foods	Foods to Avoid
- Pastries	Any product(s) that is made using or contain(s) the following:
- Pies	- Whole grains
- Sugar	- Bran
- Plain hard candy	- Coconut
- Condiments	- Nuts
- Coffee	- Seeds
- Tea	- Dried fruits
- Carbonated beverages	- Chocolate syrup
- Sherbet	- Candies made with chocolates or nuts
- Gelatine	- Horseradish
- Sponge cakes (without fruit and nuts)	
- Jelly	**More Foods to Avoid**
- Ice cream	- Cakes, puddings and biscuits made using wholemeal flour, nuts and dried fruits
- Custard	- Chocolate with dried fruit or nuts
- Semolina and rice puddings	- Toffees with dried fruit or nuts
- Jams without seeds	- Fudge with dried fruit or nuts
- Plain biscuits	- Marmalade with peel
	- Jams with seeds
	- Marzipan
	- Digestive biscuits

Chapter 4

Guidelines for Healthy Cooking

This chapter will help you with some of the standard yet important cooking guidelines that are extremely important not only for normal cooking but also for any health condition cooking too. These are basics of any kind of cooking but either people are not aware of these or do not care to follow them.

For any kind of health condition cooking, it is highly recommended that you read through each and every guideline carefully and apply them accordingly as and when required in your recipes and cooking.

How to Perfectly Measure and Weigh Ingredients

It is important for any kind of cooking that you measure your ingredients accurately. The measurement is even more important when you do cooking for certain health condition. This is required to maintain the right amount of nutrients and their nutritional values in the recipes.

The most important rules you must follow while using any cookbook are:

- Read every word of the recipe carefully.
- Make sure the measurements are accurate.

It is recommended that some sort of measuring tools are always kept in the kitchen so that they can be used as and when required. They can be of glass, plastic or even metal. Let's have a look below now what kind of measurement tools are best for measuring liquid and dry ingredients.

For liquid Ingredients

You can keep the liquid ingredients in the glass cups with pour spouts. While measuring liquid ingredients, you can simply place a cup on the flat surface and pour the liquid and read the desired mark at the eye level.

For dry ingredients

You can use individual cups in the sets of 1 cup, ½ cup, ⅓ cup and ¼ cup sizes. While measuring the dry ingredients, pile lightly into the measuring cup with spoon. Do not shake cup, level of with a straight edge.

Some Tips on measuring spoons:

- Measuring spoons are available in the sets of 1 tablespoon, 1 teaspoon, ½ teaspoon, ¼ teaspoon, and ⅛ teaspoon.
- Use for small amounts of dry foods or liquids.
- Dip spoon into dry ingredient, scoop, and then level of with a straight edge.
- Do not pour or level the ingredient over the bowl with the other ingredients.

Food Safety Guidelines

Unsafe food handling leads to food contamination and food contamination may lead to various food borne diseases such as vomiting, diarrhea, and fever. These food borne diseases occur when someone eat or drink something that is contaminated with viruses, bacteria's and parasites.

It is not common to develop a food borne disease because human immune system is strong enough to fight these harmful bacteria's but it is still a good practice to maintain the right level of hygiene and keep the food safe from being contaminated.

Keep it Separate

Raw foods like poultry, meat, fish, and seafood are some of the foods that may get contaminated very easily. Due to this fact, it is a good idea to separate these foods from others foods not only in your grocery cart but also in the refrigerator. Separating these foods from other foods will ensure that there is no cross contamination of foods.

Cross contamination is the spread of harmful viruses, parasites and bacteria's from one type of food to another. This happens when these foods come in contact with each other. Though you do cook food properly and may think that heating and cooking will kill these harmful bacteria's but the fact is, that most of the times we consume fruits and vegetables raw.

Let's take a look at some of the shopping and storage tips that may help prevent cross contamination of foods.

- While going for shopping, make sure to carry a separate bag for meat, fish, poultry and seafood.

- You can also label this bag with "Raw Meat", to avoid confusions while shopping.
- Try to pack raw foods in individual plastic bags as this will hugely avoid cross contamination.
- It is a good idea to buy cold and frozen foods always at the end.
- In the refrigerator, always store the raw meat, fish, seafood and poultry in separate containers.
- The best practice is to place the raw meat, fish, seafood and poultry in the bottom shelf of the refrigerator. This will ensure that the juices from raw meat, fish, seafood and poultry do not drip onto other foods in the refrigerator.

Keep it Clean

Apart from separating food, another important part of food safety is cleanliness. You must clean your hands, fruits, vegetables, reusable bags, utensils and kitchen surfaces thoroughly to eliminate harmful bacteria. Taking these measures will drastically help reduce the risk of one getting food borne diseases.

Let's take a look at some helpful tips to keep yourself and other stuff as clean as possible:

- Always wash your hands before touching the food with a liquid soap (preferably).
- You must wash and clean fruits and vegetables thoroughly either before eating raw or cooking.
- You must handle raw food separately. Do not use utensils that you have used to handle raw meat, fish, poultry or seafood again until you wash them thoroughly in a dishwasher or with hot soapy water.
- You must consider using paper kitchen towels instead of cloth towels. If you do use cloth towels, make sure to wash them as often as possible.

- You should consider using a vegetable scrub brush to clean vegetables with firm skin like squash, potatoes, carrots and melons etc.

This Page Has Been Left Blank Intentionally.

Chapter 5

Recipes: Main Dishes

Chicken Recipes

SPRING ONIONS AND HERBS CHICKEN CURRY

Yield	6 servings
Serving size	3-ounces

Ingredient	Quantity	Form
Whole Chicken	1	Skin removed and cut into small pieces
Lemon Juice	¼ cup	
Curry Powder	2 tsps.	
Spring Onions	½ cup	Blanched/boiled and finely chopped
Black Pepper	½ tsp.	
Thyme	½ tsp.	Dry
Vegetable Oil	2 tbsp.	
Water	1 cup	

Directions

1. Start by cleaning the whole chicken and cut into small pieces.
2. Once you cut the chicken into small pieces, give the chicken pieces a bath of lemon juice.
3. Next, take a medium sized bowl and combine spring onions, curry powder, black pepper, thyme together. Once combined, rub the mixture onto the chicken pieces.
4. Next step is to let the chicken marinate in the refrigerator overnight or at least for 1 to 2 hours.
5. Take a sauce pan and heat the vegetable oil. Sauté the marinated chicken until it turns brown.
6. Once the chicken turns brown, pour one cup of water into the pan and let the chicken simmer until it gets tender.
7. Once the chicken becomes tender, remove it from the heat and serve with hot rice.

Nutritional content per serving

Nutrition	Amount per serving
Calories	323
Trans Fat	0 grams
Sodium	93 milligrams
Protein	21 grams
Cholesterol	89 milligrams
Potassium	317 milligrams
Total Fat	24 grams
Carbohydrates	5 grams
Phosphorus	214 milligrams
Saturated Fat	6 grams
Fiber	0 grams
Calcium	25 milligrams

SPRING ONION CHICKEN

Yield	8 servings
Serving size	3-ounces

Ingredient	Quantity	Form
Vegetable Oil	3 tbsp.	
Chicken	3 pounds	Skin and fat removed, cut into pieces
Spring Onions	½ cup	Chopped
Chicken Bouillon	1 ½ cups	Low-sodium
Nutmeg	½ tsp.	Ground
Black Pepper	¼ tsp.	Ground
Cilantro	2 tsp.	Only leaves. Fresh and finely chopped

Directions

1. Start by heating the oil in a pan and brown the chicken pieces. Once the chicken pieces are brown, set them aside keeping warm.
2. In the same pan, sauté the spring onions. Now, add the chicken bouillon and bring to a boil. Keep stirring in between.
3. Once the chicken bouillon comes to a boil, add the chicken pieces, nutmeg and black pepper.
4. Cover the pan the let the chicken simmer for 30 to 35 minutes or until the chicken is tender.
5. Add cilantro to chicken and let it simmer for another minute or so. Serve hot.

Nutritional content per serving

Nutrition	Amount per serving
Calories	143
Trans Fat	0 grams
Sodium	45 milligrams
Protein	17 grams
Cholesterol	46 milligrams
Potassium	160 milligrams
Total Fat	7 grams
Carbohydrates	2 grams
Phosphorus	127 milligrams
Saturated Fat	1 gram
Fiber	0 grams
Calcium	12 milligrams

OLD STYLE RICE AND CHICKEN

Yield   6 servings
Serving size   ¾ cup

Ingredient	Quantity	Form
Chicken	1 pound	Cut into pieces
Black Pepper	½ tsp.	Ground
Poultry Seasoning	1 tbsp.	
Spring Onions	½ cup	Chopped
Onion Powder	½ tsp.	Powder form
Bay Leaves (Optional)	2-3	Crushed
Water	4 cups	
White Rice	1 cup	White and uncooked
Vegetable Oil	1 tbsp.	

Directions

1. Take a Dutch oven covered with water and put the chicken pieces, spring onions, onion powder, black pepper, poultry seasoning and bay leaves.
2. Cook the chicken until tender.
3. Once the chicken is cooked, remove the chicken meat and skin from the bone. Keep the chicken meat but discard the skin. Also reserve 2 cups of chicken broth.
4. Take a large pot and put rice, vegetable oil, chicken meat and 2 cups of chicken broth in it. Now, bring it to a boil over medium-high heat.
5. Once it comes to a boil, reduce the heat to low and simmer for about 20 to 25 minutes.
6. Serve hot.

Nutritional content per serving

Nutrition	Amount per serving
Calories	212
Trans Fat	0 grams
Sodium	76 milligrams
Protein	21 grams
Cholesterol	60 milligrams
Potassium	283 milligrams
Total Fat	8 grams
Carbohydrates	11 grams
Phosphorus	218 milligrams
Saturated Fat	2 grams
Fiber	1 gram
Calcium	25 milligrams

OVEN ROASTED LEMON AND ROSEMARY

CHICKEN

Yield   4 servings
Serving size   1/4 portion of the whole recipe

Ingredient	Quantity	Form
Butter	1 tsp.	Softened
Vegetable Oil	1 tsp.	
Rosemary	1 tsp.	Chopped
Chicken	1 (3 pounds)	
Black Pepper	1/3 tsp.	Ground
Sea Salt	1 tsp.	
Lemon	1	Cut into quarters

Directions

1. Start by preheating the oven to 450 degrees Fahrenheit.
2. Take a small bowl and mix rosemary, oil and butter together. Next, rub this mixture to the chicken thoroughly between skin and flesh.
3. Also, sprinkle a little salt and pepper inside and out of the chicken.
4. Place the chicken in a roasting pan on the bed of vegetables. Also, place a lemon inside the cavity of the chicken. Once done, tie the legs of the chicken together with a cotton string.
5. Next step is to roast the chicken for about 20 minutes.
6. After 20 minutes, reduce the temperature of the oven from 450 to 375 degrees Fahrenheit.
7. Continue to roast the chicken until the meat's thickest part of inner thigh registers 180 - 185 degrees Fahrenheit (check with a meat thermometer). Usually, this will be about 1 hour

and 15 minutes.

8. Remove the chicken from the oven. Lift and tilt the chicken to empty all the juices from the cavity.

9. Next step is to transfer the chicken to a cutting board. But wait for 10 minutes at least before carving the chicken. In the meanwhile, you can cover the chicken with an aluminium foil to keep it warm.

10. Discard vegetables.

Nutritional content per serving

Nutrition	Amount per serving
Calories	405.1
Sodium	742.0 milligrams
Protein	46.7 grams
Cholesterol	161.3 milligrams
Potassium	503.0 milligrams
Total Fat	22.6 grams
Carbohydrates	0.2 grams
Saturated Fat	6.9 gram
Fiber	0.1 grams

CHICKEN BREASTS IN BROWN SUGAR SAUCE

Yield 4 servings
Serving size 3 oz.

Ingredient	Quantity	Form
Brown Sugar	4 tsp.	
Chicken Breasts	12 ounces	Boneless and skin removed
Garlic Powder	1 tsp.	Powder form
Butter	2 tsps.	
Black Pepper	A dash	Powder form

Directions

1. Start by melting the butter in a frying pan.
2. Once the butter is melted, add the garlic powder to the pan and sauté for at least 30-40 seconds.
3. Next step is to add the chicken breasts to the pan and cook thoroughly. Add pepper to the chicken breasts and let it cook further. Repeat this step for each side of chicken breasts.
4. Once the chicken breasts are cooked, switch off the heat and add the brown sugar on top of both the breasts.
5. Let the brown sugar melt into the chicken breasts. This will take approximately 5-6 minutes. Serve hot.

Nutritional content per serving

Nutrition	Amount per serving
Calories	166.4
Sodium	87.7 milligrams

Protein	19.4 grams
Cholesterol	68.2 milligrams
Potassium	173.9 milligrams
Total Fat	8.0 grams
Carbohydrates	4.3 grams
Saturated Fat	4.2 gram
Fiber	0 grams

COLA FLAVORED CHICKEN BREASTS

Yield	3 servings
Serving size	1 chicken breast

Ingredient	Quantity	Form
Chicken Breasts	3	Boneless and skin removed
Diet Cola	1 can	
Ketchup	1 cup	

Directions

1. Start by taking a non-stick skillet and putting the chicken into it over a medium-high heat.
2. Next step is to add the diet cola of any kind and ketchup to the chicken.
3. Bring the mixture to a boil. Once it boils, reduce the heat, cover and cook for at least 40 to 45 minutes.
4. After 40 to 45 minutes, remove the cover from the skillet. Increase the heat and continue to cook until the cola sauce thickens. The sauce must stick or adhere to the chicken breasts.
5. Serve hot.

Nutritional content per serving

Nutrition	Amount per serving
Calories	159.2
Sodium	1,011.5 milligrams
Protein	16.5 grams

Cholesterol	41.2 milligrams
Potassium	188.2 milligrams
Total Fat	0.9 grams
Carbohydrates	21.4 grams
Saturated Fat	0.2 gram
Fiber	0 grams

CRISPY OVEN FRIED CHICKEN BREASTS

Yield	4 servings
Serving size	1 chicken breast

Ingredient	Quantity	Form
Chicken Breasts	4	Boneless and skin removed
Ranch Dressing Mix	1 ounce	Package
Crispy Rice Cereal	2 cups	Crushed
Parmesan Cheese	1/4 cup	Grated
Egg Whites	2	Beaten

Directions

1. Start by taking a bowl and combine the ranch mix, parmesan cheese and rice cereal together.
2. Take another small bowl or plate to pour the egg whites.
3. Next step is to dip the chicken breasts in the egg whites and then in the cereal mixture. Make sure that you coat the chicken breasts evenly.
4. Take a well-greased baking sheet and arrange the chicken breasts in it.
    Once you arrange the chicken breasts in the baking sheet, bake the chicken breasts at 375 degrees Fahrenheit until they turn golden brown. This process will take at least 30 to 35 minutes.

Nutritional content per serving

Nutrition	Amount per serving
Calories	232
Sodium	648.9 milligrams
Protein	34.4 grams
Cholesterol	84.9 milligrams
Potassium	48.7 milligrams
Total Fat	3.4 grams
Carbohydrates	15.1 grams
Saturated Fat	1.2 gram
Fiber	0.5 grams

CHICKEN AND CHEESE BALLS

Yield	8 servings
Serving size	1/8 portion of the whole recipe

Ingredient	Quantity	Form
Chicken	4 cups	Cooked and shredded
Cheddar Cheese	1 cup	Shredded
Eggs	2	
Spring Onions	1/4 cup	Chopped
Breadcrumbs	1/4 cup	Seasoned
Poultry Seasoning	2 tbsp.	

Directions

1. Start by taking a medium sized bowl and combining all the ingredients in it.
2. Place the mixture in the refrigerator and chill for at least 30 minutes.
3. Next step is to coat a large skillet with cooking spray and place it over medium high heat.
4. Take the mixture out of the refrigerator and divide into 8 equal portions. Cook these balls for approximately 5 minutes evenly until the balls are crispy and the cheese has melted.

Nutritional content per serving

Nutrition	Amount per serving
Calories	195
Sodium	194.3 milligrams
Protein	24.4 grams

Cholesterol	113.8 milligrams
Potassium	201.2 milligrams
Total Fat	8.8 grams
Carbohydrates	3.3 grams
Saturated Fat	4.1 gram
Fiber	0.2 grams

CHEESY CHICKEN BREASTS

Yield	4 servings
Serving size	1 chicken breast

Ingredient	Quantity	Form
Chicken Breasts	1	Large
Vegetable Oil	As required	
Salt	As per taste	
Pepper	As per taste	
Pasta Sauce	1 cup	
Mozzarella Cheese	8 oz.	Grated

Directions

1. Start by preheating the oven to 350° F.
2. Next step is to heat the pasta sauce in a medium sized skillet over stove.
3. Place the chicken breasts in a plastic bag and pound until they have a uniform thickness.
4. Remove the chicken breasts from the plastic bag and season with salt and pepper.
5. Next step is to take a non-stick pan and heat enough oil to sauté the chicken breasts.
6. Place the chicken breasts in the pan and sauté until they are cooked and turn golden. To be more precise, sauté for five minutes on the first side and three minutes on the other side.
7. Next step is to dip the cooked chicken breasts into the pasta sauce and then place in a casserole dish.
8. Top the chicken breasts with the remaining pasta sauce and cheese.
9. Last step is to bake the chicken breasts in the oven until the cheese is melted.

Nutritional content per serving

Nutrition	Amount per serving
Calories	349.2
Sodium	598.4 milligrams
Protein	41.9 grams
Cholesterol	101.3 milligrams
Potassium	532.9 milligrams
Total Fat	16.3 grams
Carbohydrates	6.7 grams
Saturated Fat	6.9 gram
Fiber	1 grams

PARMESAN CHICKEN BREASTS

Yield	4 servings
Serving size	1 chicken breast

Ingredient	Quantity	Form
Egg White	1	
Parmesan Cheese	¼ cup	
Cornflakes	1 ½ cup	Crushed
Salt	1/4 tsp.	
Black Pepper	1/4 tsp.	Ground
Thyme	1 tsp.	Dried
Chicken Breasts	4	Boneless and skinless

Directions

1. Start by preheating the oven to 400° F.
2. Take a small bowl and beat an egg white until it is frothy.
3. Take another bowl and combine cornflakes, salt, pepper, cheese and thyme.
4. Next step is to dip each chicken breast in the egg white and then into the cornflakes mixture. You must pat the chicken breasts well to make sure that the mixture sticks to the chicken breasts.
5. Take and pan and lightly grease it with oil.
6. Place the chicken breasts in the pan and bake for about 25 minutes or until the internal temperature of the chicken breasts reaches at least 165 degrees F.

Nutritional content per serving

Nutrition	Amount per serving
Calories	221.2
Sodium	390.2 milligrams
Protein	38.3 grams
Cholesterol	128.0 milligrams
Potassium	20.2 milligrams
Total Fat	3.2 grams
Carbohydrates	9.8 grams
Saturated Fat	1.2 gram
Fiber	0.5 grams

OVEN BROWN CRISPY LEMON CHICKEN

Yield	8 servings
Serving size	3-ounces

Ingredient	Quantity	Form
Chicken Fryer Pieces	2 ½ pound	Cut as desired
Lemon Juice	1 tbsp.	
All-Purpose Flour	1 cup	
Black Pepper	¼ teaspoon	Ground
Corn Flakes	1 cup	Crushed
Poultry Seasoning	¼ teaspoon	
Vegetable Oil	4 tbsp.	

Directions

1. Start by preheating the oven to 400ºF.
2. Next step is to wash, clean and pat dry the chicken pieces. Once the chicken pieces are dry, give them a bath of lemon juice.
3. Take a small plastic bag and combine the flour, corn flakes, black pepper and poultry seasoning together. Shake the bag well to mix the ingredients.
4. Take a deep baking pan (about 1 inch deep) and grease it with vegetable oil.
5. Put the chicken in the plastic bag of ingredients and shake well. Put the large pieces first followed by small ones.
6. Once the chicken pieces are well coated with the mixture, place them in the pan and brown in the oven for about 20 to 30 minutes on each side.

Nutritional content per serving

Nutrition	Amount per serving
Calories	280
Trans Fat	0 grams
Sodium	74 milligrams
Protein	15 grams
Cholesterol	52 milligrams
Potassium	150 milligrams
Total Fat	18 grams
Carbohydrates	15 grams
Phosphorus	120 milligrams
Saturated Fat	3 grams
Fiber	1 gram
Calcium	12 milligrams

Pork Recipes

SIMPLE 'N' BASIC PORK CHOPS

Yield   4 chops
Serving size   1 chop

Ingredient	Quantity	Form
Vegetable Oil	2 tbsp.	
All-Purpose Flour	¼ cup	
Black Pepper	1 tsp.	Ground
Sage	½ tsp.	Ground
Thyme	½ tsp.	Dried
Pork Chops	4	Lean and fat removed

Directions

1. Start by preheating the oven to 350ºF.
2. Take a baking pan and grease it well with vegetable oil.
3. Take a large bowl and combine the flour, thyme, sage and black pepper.
4. Now dredge the pork chops in the flour mixture and arrange in the baking pan.
5. Now place the baking pan into the oven and let the pork chops brown on both the sides. This process will take approximately 40-45 minutes.
6. Once the pork chops are tender, remove them from the oven and serve hot.

Nutritional content per serving

Nutrition	Amount per serving
Calories	434
Trans Fat	0 grams
Sodium	60 milligrams
Protein	19 grams
Cholesterol	79 milligrams
Potassium	332 milligrams
Total Fat	34 grams
Carbohydrates	12 grams
Phosphorus	199 milligrams
Saturated Fat	10 grams
Fiber	0 grams
Calcium	35 milligrams

SIMPLE HOMEMADE PAN PORK SAUSAGE

Yield	12 servings
Serving size	1 patty

Ingredient	Quantity	Form
Pork	1 pound	Lean and ground
Sage	2 tsp.	Ground
Sugar	2 tsp.	Granulated
Black Pepper	½ tsp.	Ground
Paprika	½ tsp.	
Basil	1 tsp.	Fresh and finely chopped
Cooking Spray		

Directions

1. Take a large bowl and mix all the ingredients well to make the sausage.
2. Once the mixture is ready, make into patties by measuring 2 tablespoons of mixture for each patty.
3. Once the patties are formed, either pan fry them or broil until they are thoroughly cooked.

Nutritional content per serving

Nutrition	Amount per serving
Calories	96
Trans Fat	0 grams
Sodium	22 milligrams
Protein	6 grams
Cholesterol	43 milligrams

Potassium	87 milligrams
Total Fat	7 grams
Carbohydrates	1 gram
Phosphorus	53 milligrams
Saturated Fat	2 grams
Fiber	0 grams
Calcium	72 milligrams

PORK CHOPS IN BROWN SUGAR & MUSTARD

Yield   6 servings
Serving size   1 pork chop

Ingredient	Quantity	Form
Pork Loin Chops	6	Boneless
Yellow Mustard	1/3 cup	
Brown Sugar	½ cup	

Directions

1. Start by preheating the oven to 350 degrees F.
2. Take a bowl and combine sugar and mustard together.
3. In a separate bowl, pour this mixture over pork chops.
4. Now arrange the pork chops in a baking tray and bake at 350 degrees F. for 25 minutes or until tender.

Nutritional content per serving

Nutrition	Amount per serving
Calories	228.1
Sodium	204.6 milligrams
Protein	20.7 grams
Cholesterol	51.1 milligrams
Potassium	375.3 milligrams
Total Fat	7.8 grams
Carbohydrates	24.6 grams
Saturated Fat	2.9 gram
Fiber	0.5 grams

GRILLED PORK TENDERLOIN

Yield	6 servings
Serving size	1 pork chop

Ingredient	Quantity	Form
Pork Chops	6	
Paprika	2 tsp.	
Oregano	1 ½ tsp.	Dried
Cumin	¾ tsp.	Ground
Garlic Powder	1/8 tsp.	Dried and powder form

Directions

1. Start by taking a small bowl and combining the oregano, paprika, cumin and garlic powder together.
2. Next step is to rub this mixture over the surface of pork chops. Once done, cover the chops and refrigerate for 24 hours. If you can't refrigerate for 24 hours, then do at least for 2 hours.
3. Remove the pork chips from the refrigerator and start grilling over medium hot coals or broil.
4. Keep turning the pork chops occasionally in between. The pork chops should be ready in approximately 15-18 minutes. Check using a meat thermometer. When the meat thermometer reads at least 155 to 160 degrees F, it means the pork chops are ready.

Nutritional content per serving

Nutrition	Amount per serving
Calories	170.7
Sodium	75.6 milligrams
Protein	28.2 grams
Cholesterol	78.3 milligrams
Potassium	480.7 milligrams
Total Fat	5.2 grams
Carbohydrates	1.4 grams
Saturated Fat	1.7 gram
Fiber	0.9 grams

OVEN SEARED PORK CHOPS

Yield	2 servings
Serving size	1 pork chop

Ingredient	Quantity	Form
Pork Chops	2	Boneless
vegetable oil	As required	
Salt	As per taste	
Pepper	As per taste	
Spices	(See the recipe)	

Directions

1. Start by preheating the oven to 450° F.
2. Take a heavy, oven proof skillet and heat it over medium-high heat.
3. Take a bowl and coat the pork chops well with oil.
4. Now season the pork chops with salt, pepper and spices. Some of the best spices that can be used in this recipe are coriander powder, garlic powder and cumin. Please use the garlic powder in moderation.
5. Now, place the pork chops into the pan and sear them on each side for about 2 to 3 minutes or until golden in colour.
6. Once the pork chops turn golden, remove the skillet from heat and place it inside the oven and cook until the pork chops are cooked thoroughly.
7. Once the pork chops are cooked thoroughly, remove from oven and let them rest for about 5 to 10 minutes before serving.

Nutritional content per serving

Nutrition	Amount per serving
Calories	322.0
Sodium	248.6 milligrams
Protein	39.0 grams
Cholesterol	111.9 milligrams
Potassium	514.1 milligrams
Total Fat	17.3 grams
Carbohydrates	0.1 grams
Saturated Fat	5.1 gram
Fiber	0 grams

Lamb Recipes

GINGER & MUSTARD LAMB

Yield	4 servings
Serving size	3-ounces

Ingredient	Quantity	Form
Vegetable Oil	¼ cup	
Ginger Powder	1 ½ tbsp.	Powder form
Mustard	3 tsp.	Dry
Leg Of Lamb	1	Trimmed for roasting purpose

Directions

1. Start by taking a medium sized bowl and combining oil, mustard and ginger powder together well.
2. Now, put and coat the lamb legs well with the mixture. Once the lamb legs are coated well with mixture, refrigerate the lamb legs for at least 6 to 8 hours or overnight.
3. Remove the lamb from refrigerate and place on barbeque spit.
4. Keep basting the meat continuously with the marinade and roast the lamb legs for around 30 minutes or until the meat thermometer reads the temperature of the lamb at 170 degrees F.

Nutritional content per serving

Nutrition	Amount per serving
Calories	289
Trans Fat	0 grams

Sodium	144 milligrams
Protein	24 grams
Cholesterol	73 milligrams
Potassium	423 milligrams
Total Fat	6 grams
Carbohydrates	3 grams
Phosphorus	237 milligrams
Saturated Fat	2 grams
Fiber	0 grams
Calcium	14 milligrams

AROMATIC LAMB CHOPS

| **Yield** | 4 servings |
| **Serving size** | 3 lamb chops |

Ingredient	Quantity	Form
Lemon Juice	1/4 cup	Fresh
Lemon Juice	2 tbsp.	Fresh
Rosemary	3 tbsp.	Fresh and chopped
Garlic Powder	½ tsp.	Powder form
Salt	1/4 tsp.	
Pepper	1/4 tsp.	
Lamb Chops	12	

Directions

1. Start by preheating the broiler on high heat.
2. Take a bowl and combining rosemary, lemon juice, garlic powder, salt and pepper together.
3. Now, rub this mixture on the lamb chops well and evenly. Once the lamb chops are coated with the mixture set them aside on a plate.
4. Take a cast iron or stainless steel skillet which is large enough to hold the lamb chops and place in the broiler under the heat to become very hot. Place the skillet about 5 to 7 inches from the heat source. Also make sure that the handle of the skillet is also made of metal.
5. Once the skillet is hot, place the lamb chops in the skillet and return to the broiler for approximately 4 to 5 minutes or depending on the thickness of the lamb. Lamb will cook fast as it is cooking on both the sides at the same time.

Nutritional content per serving

Nutrition	Amount per serving
Calories	234.7
Sodium	259.8 milligrams
Protein	35.0 grams
Cholesterol	108.9 milligrams
Potassium	624.2 milligrams
Total Fat	8.5 grams
Carbohydrates	2.6 grams
Saturated Fat	3.4 gram
Fiber	0.4 grams

MUSTARD LAMB CHOPS

Yield	4 servings
Serving size	2 lamb chops

Ingredient	Quantity	Form
Lamb chops	8	1 ½ inches
Mustard	2 tbsp.	Dijon style
Vegetable oil	1 tbsp.	
Rosemary	1 tbsp.	Chopped
Black pepper	1/8 tsp.	Ground

Directions

1. Start by preheating the broiler. You need to add ½ inch water to the broiler pan in order to prevent the smoking. Set aside.
2. Next step is to combine the rosemary, mustard oil and pepper in a small bowl. Once the mustard mixture is ready, brush both sides of the lamb chops with mustard mixture and place the chops on the unheated broiler pan.
3. Next step is to broil the chops (4 inches from the heat) until desired doneness achieved, turning once.
4. Serve immediately.

Nutritional content per serving

Nutrition	Amount per serving
Calories	262.6
Sodium	767.6 milligrams
Protein	17.3 grams
Cholesterol	53.9 milligrams

Potassium	302.6 milligrams
Total Fat	18.1 grams
Carbohydrates	0.5 grams
Saturated Fat	3.7 grams
Fiber	0.3 grams

HERBACEOUS LAMB CHOPS

Yield   3 servings
Serving size   1 lamb chop

Ingredient	Quantity	Form
Lamb Chops	3	1 inch thick and excess fat removed
Mustard	1 tbsp.	Dijon
Basil	2 tbsp.	Fresh and finely chopped
Rosemary	1 tbsp.	Fresh and finely chopped
Oregano	1 tbsp.	Dried and crushed
Salt	As per taste	
Black Pepper	As per taste	Ground

Directions

1. Start by preheating the oven to 375° F.
2. Next step is to chop the herbs finely. Once chopped, add salt and pepper to the herbs. Once done, spread the herbs evenly on the chopping board.
3. Next step is to rub the chops with Dijon. Rub one teaspoon of Dijon per chop.
4. Now, take one chop at a time and coat with the herbs on all the sides. Once coated, shake the chop to remove excess herbs.
5. Next step is to place the chops in the baking pan (big enough to hold all the chops without chops touching each other)
6. Now, roast the chops in the preheated oven for about 15 minutes for medium rare. If you want the medium doneness, roast for slightly longer peroid.

Nutritional content per serving

Nutrition	Amount per serving
Calories	133.7
Sodium	320.2 milligrams
Protein	18.6 grams
Cholesterol	57.6 milligrams
Potassium	344.7 milligrams
Total Fat	4.6 grams
Carbohydrates	1.2 grams
Saturated Fat	1.8 grams
Fiber	0.8 grams

GRILLED LAMB CHOPS

Yield	4 servings
Serving size	1 lamb chop

Ingredient	Quantity	Form
Lamb Chops	4, 4 oz.	
Garlic Powder	1/2 tsp.	Powder form
Rosemary	1 tbsp.	Fresh and minced
Vegetable Oil	2 tbsp.	

Directions

1. Start by taking a medium bowl and mixing all the ingredients, except the lamb chops.
2. Next step is to rub both the sides of each lamb chop with the mixture. Once done, let the chops sit for at least 30 minutes or overnight.
3. Before starting the grilling, salt and pepper both sides of lamb chops as per the taste.
4. Now, grill the lamb chops to the desired doneness.

Nutritional content per serving

Nutrition	Amount per serving
Calories	214.4
Sodium	73.2 milligrams
Protein	23.4 grams
Cholesterol	72.6 milligrams
Potassium	402.7 milligrams
Total Fat	12.4 grams

Carbohydrates	1.1 grams
Saturated Fat	3.1 grams
Fiber	0.1 grams

Beef Recipes

BEEF STEAK WITH CARROTS AND MINT

Yield   4 servings
Serving size   3 oz. steak, ½ Cup salad

Ingredient for Steak	Quantity	Form
Beef Top Sirloin Steaks	4 (3 oz. per steak)	
Salt	¼ tsp.	
Black Pepper	¼ tsp.	Ground
Vegetable Oil	½ tbsp.	

Ingredient for Salad	Quantity	Form
Carrots	1 cup	Skinless. Well blanched or boiled, rinsed and grated
Cucumber	1 cup	Skinless. Well blanched or boiled, rinsed, peeled and sliced
Vegetable Oil	1 tbsp.	
Mint	2 tbsp.	Fresh and rinsed. Shredded
Salt	¼ tsp.	
Black Pepper	¼ tsp.	Ground
Orange Juice	½ cup	Without bits

Directions for Steak

1.   Start by preheating the grill pan or the oven broiler (with the

rack 3 inches from the heat source) on high temperature.
2. *Prepare the salad. Please find the steps in the next table.*
3. Next step is to lightly coat the steak with oil and season with salt and pepper.
4. Now, grill or broil the steak, 2 to 3 minutes on each side or until desired doneness is achieved. For the best results, the internal temperature of the steak should not exceed 145 ºF.
5. Once the steak is done, remove it from the heat and allow it to cool for about 5 minutes.
6. Now, serve one 3 ounces steak with about ½ cup of salad.

Directions for Salad

1. Combine all the salad ingredients in a bowl and mix gently. Allow all the flavours to blend for at least 10 to 15 minutes.

Nutritional content per serving

Nutrition	Amount per serving
Calories	191
Sodium	359 milligrams
Protein	19 grams
Cholesterol	35 milligrams
Potassium	451 milligrams
Total Fat	9 grams
Carbohydrates	9 grams
Saturated Fat	2 gram
Fiber	1 grams

HERBS BEEF BURGER

Yield	4 servings
Serving size	1 patty, 3-ounces

Ingredient	Quantity	Form
Beef	1 pound	Lean and ground
Lemon Juice	1 tbsp.	Fresh
Parsley	1 tbsp.	Flakes
Black Pepper	¼ tsp.	Ground
Thyme	¼ tsp.	Ground
Oregano	¼ tsp.	Dried

Directions

1. Start by mixing all the ingredients thoroughly in a medium or large bowl.
2. Next step is to shape the mixture into patties. Please make the patties about ¾ inches thick.
3. Now, take a skillet or broiler pan and grease it with a little oil.
4. Final step is to broil the patties about 3 inches from the heat for about 10 to 15 minutes, turning once.

Nutritional content per serving

Nutrition	Amount per serving
Calories	171
Trans Fat	0 grams
Sodium	108 milligrams
Protein	20 grams
Cholesterol	90 milligrams

Potassium	289 milligrams
Total Fat	10 grams
Carbohydrates	0 grams
Phosphorus	180 milligrams
Saturated Fat	3 grams
Fiber	0 grams
Calcium	21 milligrams

HOMEMADE BEEF MEATBALLS

Yield 35 meatballs
Serving size 2 meatballs

Ingredient for Meatballs	Quantity	Form
Beef	1 pound	Lean and ground
Spring Onions	¼ cup	Finely chopped
Lemon Juice	1 tbsp.	
Poultry Seasoning	1 tsp.	Without salt
Black Pepper	1tsp.	Ground
Mustard	¼ tsp.	Dry
Onion Powder	¾ tsp.	Powder form
Italian Seasoning	1 tsp.	
Sugar	1 tsp.	Granulated

Ingredient for Sauce	Quantity	Form
Vegetable Oil	¼ cup	
All-Purpose Flour	2 tbsp.	
Onion Powder	1 tsp.	Powder form
Vinegar	2 tsp.	
Sugar	2 tsp.	
Some Mild Sauce For Flavour	1 tsp.	Avoid chilli sauce
Water	2-3 cups	

Directions for Sauce

1. Start by taking a sauce pan, placing on heat and combining oil and flour in it. Keep stirring.
2. Now, add vinegar, sugar, onion powder, mild sauce and water

3. Once you add all the ingredients, return the pan to heat and continue stirring until the sauce thickens.

Directions for Meatballs

1. Start by preheating the oven to 425ºF.
2. Next step is to take a bowl and mix all the ingredients together well.
3. Once the mixture is ready, shape the meatballs. Each meatball should have one tablespoon of meat mixture.
4. Now, place the meatballs in a baking dish and bake them for about 20 minutes or until well done.
5. Final step is to remove the meatballs from the oven and combine them with the sauce. Keep the meatballs warm until you are ready to serve.

Nutritional content per serving

Nutrition	Amount per serving
Calories	76
Trans Fat	0 grams
Sodium	31 milligrams
Protein	5 grams
Cholesterol	21 milligrams
Potassium	70 milligram
Total Fat	6 grams
Carbohydrates	2 grams
Phosphorus	44 milligrams
Saturated Fat	1 grams
Fiber	0 grams
Calcium	7 milligrams

BEEF STEAK SANDWICH

Yield   4 servings
Serving size   3-ounces

Ingredient	Quantity	Form
Beef Steak	4 (4 ounces each)	Chopped
Lemon Juice	1 tbsp.	
Italian Seasoning	1 tbsp.	
Black Pepper	1 tbsp.	Ground
Vegetable Oil	1 tbsp.	
White Bread Slices	4	Dry roasted in a pan
Spring Onions	½ cup	Chopped

Directions

1. Start by taking a bowl and combining the meat, Italian seasoning, black pepper and lemon juice in it.
2. Next step is to take a frying pan and heat the oil over medium heat.
3. Next step is to brown the beef steaks on both the sides until they are tender. Once done, remove from the pan and drain on the paper towels.
4. Now, reduce the heat and in the same pan, add onions and sauté them until they are tender.
5. In order to serve, serve open faced on roasted or grilled bread slices.

Nutritional content per serving

Nutrition	Amount per serving
Calories	345
Trans Fat	0 grams
Sodium	247 milligrams
Protein	14 grams
Cholesterol	40 milligrams
Potassium	200 milligrams
Total Fat	21 grams
Carbohydrates	26 grams
Phosphorus	115 milligrams
Saturated Fat	7 grams
Fiber	2 grams
Calcium	98 milligrams

Turkey Recipes

SIMPLE 'N' BASIC TURKEY MEAT LOAF

Yield	8 servings
Serving size	2-ounces

Ingredient	Quantity	Form
Turkey	1 pound	Lean and ground
Egg White	1	
Lemon Juice	1 tbsp.	
White Bread Crumbs	½ cup	Plain
Onion Powder	½ tsp.	Powder form
Italian Seasoning	½ tsp.	
Black Pepper	¼ tsp.	Ground
Spring Onions	¼ cup	Finely chopped
Water	¼ cup	

Directions

1. Start by preheating the oven to 400ºF.
2. Place the meat in a bowl and pour lemon juice on it.
3. Add all other remaining ingredients to meat and mix well.
4. Finally, place the loaf in a pan and bake for about 45 minutes.

Nutritional content per serving

Nutrition	Amount per serving
Calories	110
Trans Fat	0 grams
Sodium	71 milligrams
Protein	12 grams

Cholesterol	42 milligrams
Potassium	138 milligrams
Total Fat	5 grams
Carbohydrates	2 grams
Phosphorus	87 milligrams
Saturated Fat	1 grams
Fiber	0 grams
Calcium	20 milligram

Seafood Recipes

FISH CROQUETTES

Yield	8 patties
Serving size	1 patty

Ingredient	Quantity	Form
Salmon Or Tuna	1 can water packed	
Egg Whites	2	
Spring Onions	¼ cup	Finely chopped
Black Pepper	½ tsp.	Ground
White Bread Crumbs	½ cup	Plain
Vegetable Oil	1 tbsp.	
Lemon Juice	2 tbsps.	Fresh

Directions

1. Start by draining the water from the canned meat.
2. Next step is to take a medium bowl and combine all the ingredients except oil and mix well.
3. Once the mixture is mixed well, form the mixture into 8 separate balls, and then flatten them to form patties.
4. Next step is to take a skillet and heat vegetable oil in it.
5. Once the oil is hot, place the patties in it.
6. Brown the patties on each side. Once the patties are cooked, drain them on paper towels.

Nutritional content per serving

Nutrition	Amount per serving
Calories	189
Trans Fat	0 grams
Sodium	337 milligrams
Protein	14 grams
Cholesterol	81 milligrams
Potassium	184 milligrams
Total Fat	8 grams
Carbohydrates	11 grams
Phosphorus	191 milligrams
Saturated Fat	2 grams
Fiber	1 gram
Calcium	124 milligrams

BAKED TROUT FILLETS

Yield	4 servings
Serving size	3-ounces

Ingredient	Quantity	Form
Trout Filets	4, 3-ounce	
Black Pepper	1 ½ tsp.	Ground
Garlic Powder	1 tbsp.	Powder form
Paprika	1 ½ tsp.	
Spring Onions	¼ cup	Finely chopped
Lemon	1	Small
Parmesan Cheese	2 tbsps.	

Directions

1. Start by preheating the oven to 375ºF.
2. Next step is to place the fish in a greased baking pan or on aluminium foil.
3. Now sprinkle the garlic powder, black pepper, and paprika on both sides of the fish.
4. Also place the chopped spring onions on fish.
5. Now, squeeze the juice of one lemon onto fish.
6. It's now time to bake the fish for 30 minutes.
7. After the fish has cooked, sprinkle with parmesan cheese. Serve hot.

Nutritional content per serving

Nutrition	Amount per serving
Calories	164
Trans Fat	0 grams
Sodium	86 milligrams
Protein	20 grams
Cholesterol	62 milligrams
Potassium	452 milligrams
Total Fat	6 grams
Carbohydrates	8 grams
Phosphorus	252 milligrams
Saturated Fat	1 grams
Fiber	3 grams
Calcium	80 milligrams

BAKED LEMON CRAB CAKES

Yield	4 servings
Serving size	1 patty

Ingredient	Quantity	Form
Egg	1	
Crackers	½ cup	Low sodium
Mayonnaise	¼ cup	Reduced fat
Mustard	1 tbsp.	Dry
Black Pepper	1 tsp.	Ground
Lemon Juice	2 tbsps.	Fresh
Garlic Powder	1 tsp.	Powder form
Vegetable Oil	2 tbsps.	

Directions

1. Start by combining all ingredients.
2. Now, divide the mixture into 6 balls and form patties.
3. Take a pan and heat vegetable oil at medium heat or oven at 350ºF.
4. Fry the patties for about 4-5 minutes or bake in the oven for 15 minutes.
5. Serve warm.

Nutritional content per serving

Nutrition	Amount per serving
Calories	101
Trans Fat	0 grams
Sodium	67 milligrams

Protein	2 grams
Cholesterol	41 milligrams
Potassium	72 milligrams
Total Fat	9 grams
Carbohydrates	5 grams
Phosphorus	43 milligrams
Saturated Fat	1 gram
Fiber	0 grams
Calcium	16 milligrams

BAKED FLAKY FISH FILLETS

Yield	4 servings
Serving size	3 ½-ounces

Ingredient	Quantity	Form
Fish Filets	12-16	Tilapia or as desired
Saltine Crackers	20	Unsalted tops and finely crushed
Butter	¼ cup	Unsalted
Dill Weed	2 tsp.	
Garlic Powder	1 tsp.	Powder form
Lemon Juice	¼ cup	Fresh

Directions

1. Start by preheating the oven to 400ºF.
2. Now, combine the dill, crackers and garlic powder.
3. Next, melt the butter or margarine.
4. Now, roll the fish in the melted butter, then in crumbs and again in the butter mix.
5. Finally, place in the baking pan and bake for about 8 to 10 minutes until the fish is flaky.

Nutritional content per serving

Nutrition	Amount per serving
Calories	164
Trans Fat	0 grams
Sodium	138 milligrams
Protein	21 grams

Cholesterol	57 milligrams
Potassium	335 milligrams
Total Fat	6 grams
Carbohydrates	7 grams
Phosphorus	181 milligrams
Saturated Fat	4 grams
Fiber	0 grams
Calcium	23 milligrams

Egg Recipes

HERBACEOUS OMELETTE

Yield	2 servings
Serving size	½ omelette

Ingredient	Quantity	Form
Vegetable Oil	1 ½ tsps.	
Spring Onions	¼ cup	Finely chopped
Eggs	4	
Water	2 tbsps.	
Basil	¼ tsp.	Dry
Tarragon	⅛ tsp.	Dry
Parsley	¼ tsp.	Dry

Directions

1. Take a bowl and beat the eggs. Now, add water and spices.
2. Now, heat the oil in an 8" frying pan over medium heat. Once the oil is hot, add and sauté the spring onions. Remove from the pan.
3. Now, pour the mixture into heated frying pan over medium heat.
4. As the omelette sets, lift with the help of a spatula to let the uncooked portion of the omelette flow to the bottom.
5. When the omelette is completely set, add the sautéed spring onions to the top of the omelette and remove from pan to a serving dish.

Nutritional content per serving

Nutrition	Amount per serving
Calories	195
Trans Fat	0 grams
Sodium	157 milligrams
Protein	14 grams
Cholesterol	474 milligrams
Potassium	157 milligrams
Total Fat	15 gram
Carbohydrates	0 grams
Phosphorus	214 milligrams
Saturated Fat	4 grams
Fiber	0 grams
Calcium	60 milligrams

This Page Has Been Left Blank Intentionally.

Chapter 6

Recipes: Sides Dishes

Rice Recipes

WHITE RICE O'BRIEN

Yield   4 servings
Serving size   ½ cup

Ingredient	Quantity	Form
Water	1½ cup	
White rice	1 cup	Uncooked
Spring onion	½ cup	Finely chopped
Carrots	¼ cup	Shredded
Paprika	¼ tsp.	
Black pepper	½ tsp.	Ground
Thyme	½ tsp.	Dry
Lemon juice	1 tbsp.	Fresh
Margarine	1 tbsp.	

Directions

1. Take a large saucepan and boil water in it. In the boiling water, combine all ingredients.
2. Cover the pan and let it simmer for about 15 minutes without stirring.
3. Now, remove from the pan and fluff the rice lightly with the help of a fork.

Nutritional content per serving

Nutrition	Amount per serving
Calories	207
Trans Fat	1 gram
Sodium	32 milligrams

Protein	4 grams
Cholesterol	0 milligrams
Potassium	125 milligrams
Total Fat	3 grams
Carbohydrates	40 grams
Phosphorus	64 milligrams
Saturated Fat	1 grams
Fiber	1 grams
Calcium	21 milligrams

HERBS & VEGGIES RICE CASSEROLE

Yield	8 servings
Serving size	½ cup

Ingredient	Quantity	Form
White Rice	1 cup	Uncooked
Chicken Stock	2 cups	Unsalted
Zucchini	½ cup	Skinless. Fresh and finely chopped
Carrots	½ cup	Skinless. Fresh and finely chopped
Parsley	½ tsp.	Flakes
Vegetable Oil	1 tbsp.	
Spring Onions	½ cup	Finely chopped
Chives	1 tbsp.	Dry

Directions

1. Start by preheating the oven to 350ºF.
2. Next step is to combine all the ingredients and place in casserole dish.
3. Finally, bake in a covered casserole for about 45 to 50 minutes or until the liquid is absorbed.

Nutritional content per serving

Nutrition	Amount per serving
Calories	53
Trans Fat	0 grams
Sodium	19 milligrams

Protein	2 grams
Cholesterol	0 milligrams
Potassium	74 milligrams
Total Fat	2 grams
Carbohydrates	7 grams
Phosphorus	29 milligrams
Saturated Fat	0 grams
Fiber	0 grams
Calcium	7 milligrams

CHICKEN BREASTS ON WHITE RICE

Yield	3 servings
Serving size	1/3 portion of whole recipe

Ingredient	Quantity	Form
Chicken Breasts	3	Skin removed
Campbell's Cream Soup	1 can	Chicken with herb
White Rice	2 cups	Cooked
Milk	1/2 cup	2%

Directions

1. Take a pan and place the chicken in it. Now, pour the rice, soup, and milk over the chicken.
2. Cover the pan with foil and bake at 350 degrees for about 45-50 minutes.

Nutritional content per serving

Nutrition	Amount per serving
Calories	233.4
Sodium	793.4 milligrams
Protein	19.5 grams
Cholesterol	53.4 milligrams
Potassium	181.0 milligrams
Total Fat	5.4 grams
Carbohydrates	24.3 grams
Saturated Fat	2.1 gram
Fiber	0.3 grams

SIMPLE MEXICAN RICE

Yield	8 servings
Serving size	1/8 portion of whole recipe

Ingredient	Quantity	Form
Vegetable Oil	2 tbsp.	
White Rice	1 ½ cups	Uncooked
Tomato Sauce	1 cup	
Water	2 cups	
Chicken Bouillon Cubes	3	Crushed
Onion Powder	As per taste	

Directions

1. Take a large saucepan and brown the rice in oil.
2. While the rice browns, combine together water, tomato sauce, chicken bouillon, and a couple sprinkles of the onion powder.
3. Now, cover and bring it to a boil, reduce the heat and let simmer until the liquid is absorbed (about 25 minutes).

Nutritional content per serving

Nutrition	Amount per serving
Calories	83.1
Sodium	449.8 milligrams
Protein	1.5 grams
Cholesterol	0.2 milligrams
Potassium	120.6 milligrams

Total Fat	3.7 grams
Carbohydrates	11.1 grams
Saturated Fat	0.5 grams
Fiber	0.6 grams

SIMPLE SPANISH RICE

Yield	6 servings
Serving size	1/6 portion of whole recipe

Ingredient	Quantity	Form
Canola Oil	2 tbsp.	
White Rice	1 cup	Long grain and uncooked
Water	2 cups	
Salt	1 tsp.	
Chicken Bouillon	2 tsp.	Seasoning
Tomato Sauce	½ cup	No chilli

Directions

1. Take a medium sized metallic skillet and brown 1 cup of white rice with oil. While browning, make sure not to brown the rice too much. The rice should just turn barely golden in colour.
2. Now, add 2 cups of water along with 1/2 cup of tomato sauce once the rice has browned a bit.
3. Now, add the bouillon seasonings and salt.
4. Cover the skillet and let simmer for about 20 minutes.

Nutritional content per serving

Nutrition	Amount per serving
Calories	162.0
Sodium	1,070.2 milligrams
Protein	2.5 grams

Cholesterol	0.0 milligrams
Potassium	103.2 milligrams
Total Fat	5.0 grams
Carbohydrates	26.3 grams
Saturated Fat	0.4 grams
Fiber	0.7 grams

Breads & Other Starches Recipes

EASY ZUCCHINI BREAD

Yield   14 servings
Serving size   1 slice

Ingredient	Quantity	Form
Zucchini	1 cup	Skinless. Grated
Sugar	1 cup	
Egg	1	
Canola Oil	¼ cup	
All-Purpose Flour	1 ½ cup	
Cinnamon	1 tsp.	Ground
Baking Soda	½ tsp.	
Nutmeg	½ tsp.	Ground
Baking Powder	¼ tsp.	
Salt	½ tsp.	

Directions

1. Start by beating together the zucchini, egg and sugar. Add oil and mix well.
2. Next step is to stir together the flour, baking soda, baking powder, cinnamon, nutmeg, and 1/2 teaspoon salt. Stir into zucchini mixture.
3. Now, pour the mixture into a greased loaf pan and bake at 350 until done. This will take about 30 to 40 minutes.
4. Make sure to cool thoroughly on rack.
5. Once cool, wrap and store overnight before slicing.

Nutritional content per serving

Nutrition	Amount per serving
Calories	147.4
Sodium	142.0 milligrams
Protein	1.9 grams
Cholesterol	15.2 milligrams
Potassium	63.4 milligrams
Total Fat	4.4 grams
Carbohydrates	25.4 grams
Saturated Fat	0.4 gram
Fiber	0.7 grams

EASY LEMON BREAD

Yield   16 servings
Serving size   1 slice

Ingredient	Quantity	Form
All-Purpose Flour	1 ¾ cup	
Sugar	¾ cup	White
Baking Powder	2 tsp.	
Salt	¼ tsp.	
Egg Whites	2	
Milk	1 cup	No fat
Applesauce	¼ cup	Unsweetened
Lemon Peel	2 tbsp.	Extremely finely shredded
Lemon Juice	1 tbsp.	Fresh

Directions

1. Start by preheat the oven to 350 degrees.
2. Take an 8x4x2 inches loaf pan and spray it lightly with cooking oil.
3. Take a medium bowl and combine the flour, baking powder, sugar, and salt. Now, make a well in the center of flour mixture and set aside.
4. Take another medium bowl and combine the egg whites, milk, lemon peel, applesauce, and lemon juice.
5. Now, add the egg mixture all at once to the flour mixture. Stir just until moistened. The batter should be quite lumpy. Now, spread the batter into the prepared loaf pan.
6. Finally, bake for about 50 to 55 minutes or until wooden toothpick inserted near center comes out clean.

Nutritional content per serving

Nutrition	Amount per serving
Calories	114.3
Sodium	76.0 milligrams
Protein	3.2 grams
Cholesterol	0.3 milligrams
Potassium	59.5 milligrams
Total Fat	1.8 grams
Carbohydrates	21.7 grams
Saturated Fat	0.1 grams
Fiber	0.7 grams

SIMPLY OLD STYLE PANCAKES

Yield   4 small pancakes
Serving size   1 pancake

Ingredient	Quantity	Form
All-Purpose Flour	½ cup	
Egg	1	Beaten
Sugar	¼ cup	Granulated
Baking Powder	¼ tsp.	
Milk	¼ cup	2% milk
Water	¼ cup	
Vegetable Oil	1 tbsp.	

Directions

1. Take a bowl and combine the first four ingredients. Mix them well.
2. Now, add water and milk. For thinner pancakes, add more water or for thicker pancakes, less water.
3. Now, take a griddle or skillet and heat oil.
4. Pour ¼ cup of batter on the griddle and cook until the pan cake is brown, turning on each side.

Nutritional content per serving

Nutrition	Amount per serving
Calories	165
Trans Fat	0 grams
Sodium	58 milligrams
Protein	4 grams

Cholesterol	61 milligrams
Potassium	57 milligrams
Total Fat	5 grams
Carbohydrates	26 grams
Phosphorus	64 milligrams
Saturated Fat	1 gram
Fiber	0 grams
Calcium	45 milligram

THE FRENCH TOAST

Yield	4 servings
Serving size	1 slice

Ingredient	Quantity	Form
Egg Whites	4	Large and slightly beaten
Milk	¼ cup	1%
Cinnamon	½ tsp.	Ground
Allspice	¼ tsp.	Ground
White Bread	4	Slices, toasted
Margarine	1 tbsp.	

Directions

1. Start by adding milk, allspice and cinnamon to the egg whites.
2. Now, dip the bread into the batter, one piece at a time.
3. Now, place the bread on a heated grill or in a skillet with melted margarine.
4. Turn the bread once turns golden brown.
5. To Serve: serve hot with sugar free syrup.

Nutritional content per serving

Nutrition	Amount per serving
Calories	125
Trans Fat	0 grams
Sodium	194 milligrams
Protein	7 grams
Cholesterol	0 milligrams
Potassium	128 milligrams

Total Fat	5 grams
Carbohydrates	14 grams
Phosphorus	61 milligrams
Saturated Fat	0 grams
Fiber	1 gram
Calcium	60 milligrams

THE DINNER ROLLS

Yield   20 servings
Serving size 1 roll

Ingredient	Quantity	Form
Water	1 cup	Hot
Vegetable Shortening	6 tbsps.	
Sugar	½ cup	
Yeast	1 package	
Water	2 tbsps.	Warm
Egg	1	
All-Purpose Flour	3 ¾-4 cups	

Directions

1. Start by preheating the oven to 400ºF.
2. Take a large bowl and combine hot water, sugar and shortening. Now keep aside to cool to the room temperature.
3. Now, dissolve the yeast in warm water.
4. Next step is to take a large bowl and add the egg, half the flour and yeast. Beat the mixture well.
5. Now, stir in remaining flour with a spoon, until it's easy to handle.
6. Now, place the dough in a greased bowl; grease top and cover top with plastic wrap.
7. Allow to rest for about 1 to 1 ½ hours or until the dough has doubled in size.
8. Cut the amount of dough needed to shape the rolls.
9. Finally, bake the rolls for about 12 minutes or until done.

Nutritional content per serving

Nutrition	Amount per serving
Calories	148
Trans Fat	0 grams
Sodium	5 milligrams
Protein	3 grams
Cholesterol	12 milligrams
Potassium	31 milligrams
Total Fat	4 grams
Carbohydrates	24 grams
Phosphorus	32 milligrams
Saturated Fat	1 grams
Fiber	1 gram
Calcium	5 milligrams

Vegetables Recipes

STEAMED FRESH ASPARAGUS

Yield	4 servings
Serving size	3 spears

Ingredient	Quantity	Form
Lemon Juice	1 tbsp.	
Margarine	2 tbsps.	Melted and unsalted
Water	2 cups	
Asparagus Spears	12	Fresh and young

Directions

1. Start by adding the lemon juice to the margarine and set aside.
2. Now, bring the water to a boil in bottom of steamer.
3. Place the asparagus in the steamer over boiling water.
4. Now, steam for about 2 to 4 minutes after the asparagus turns bright green. Please make sure that the asparagus is either well or soft cooked.
5. Now, remove and pour the margarine with lemon juice over asparagus and serve.

Nutritional content per serving

Nutrition	Amount per serving
Calories	62
Trans Fat	0 grams
Sodium	1 milligram
Protein	1 gram
Cholesterol	0 milligrams
Potassium	123 milligrams
Total Fat	6 grams

Carbohydrates	3 grams
Phosphorus	32 milligrams
Saturated Fat	1 gram
Fiber	1 gram
Calcium	16 milligrams

SPRING ONIONS & SQUASH

Yield	3 servings
Serving size	½ cup

Ingredient	Quantity	Form
Squash	2 cups	Crook neck or yellow straight neck, washed and sliced
Margarine	2 tbsps.	
Spring Onion	1 cup	Chopped
Black Pepper	1 tsp.	Ground

Directions

1. Start by boiling the squash slices for about 15 minutes or until tender. Drain.
2. Take a frying pan and melt the butter. Sauté the spring onions for about one minute.
3. Now, stir in the squash and black pepper.
4. Cover the pan and allow it to simmer on low heat for about 5 minutes.
5. Serve hot.

Nutritional content per serving

Nutrition	Amount per serving
Calories	87
Trans Fat	1 gram
Sodium	347 milligrams
Protein	1.5 gram

Cholesterol	0 milligrams
Potassium	204 milligrams
Total Fat	8 grams
Carbohydrates	4 grams
Phosphorus	40 milligrams
Saturated Fat	2 grams
Fiber	2 grams
Calcium	31 milligrams

VEGGIES QUICHE

Yield	6 servings
Serving size	1/6 portion of whole recipe

Ingredient	Quantity	Form
Bisquick	½ cup	Fat reduced
Carrots	¾ cup	Skinless. Chopped and drained
Zucchini	¾ cup	Skinless. Chopped and drained
Cheddar Cheese	1 cup	Fat reduced
Egg Beaters	1 cup	
Milk	1 ½ cup	Evaporated skim
Salt	As per taste	
Pepper	As per taste	Ground
Nutmeg	A dash	Powder

Directions

1. Start by mixing eggs, Bisquick and evaporated milk.
2. Now, fold in the zucchini and carrots.
3. Now, fold in the shredded reduced fat cheese.
4. Add a dash of salt, nutmeg powder and pepper.
5. Pour the mixture into a pan prepared with non-stick cooking spray.
6. Finally, bake at 350°F for about 40 to 50 minutes in a pie plate or an 8x8 pan.

Nutritional content per serving

Nutrition	Amount per serving
Calories	165.2
Sodium	398.7 milligrams
Protein	16.4 grams
Cholesterol	7.6 milligrams
Potassium	433.4 milligrams
Total Fat	3.8 grams
Carbohydrates	16.2 grams
Saturated Fat	1.3 gram
Fiber	0.6 grams

SIMPLY BEETS

Yield	4 servings
Serving size	1/4 portion of whole recipe

Ingredient	Quantity	Form
Beets	16 ounce	Can
Beet Liquid	½ cup	
Vinegar	½ cup	
Potato Starch	4 tsps.	
Sugar Substitute	Equivalent of 2 tbsps. of sugar	
Salt	A pinch	

Directions

1. Start by draining the beets, reserving about 1/2 cup of liquid.
2. Take a medium saucepan and combine all the ingredients.
3. Next step is to cook and stir over medium heat until the beets are cooked and soft.

Nutritional content per serving

Nutrition	Amount per serving
Calories	44.8
Sodium	219.0 milligrams
Protein	0.4 grams
Cholesterol	0.0 milligrams
Potassium	113.8 milligrams
Total Fat	0.0 grams

Carbohydrates	10.3 grams
Saturated Fat	0.0 grams
Fiber	0.9 grams

SWEET BEETS IN BUTTER

Yield	10 servings
Serving size	1/10 portion of whole recipe

Ingredient	Quantity	Form
Beets	1 bunch	
Sugar	1/3 cup	
Salt	¼ tsp.	
Potato Starch	1 tsp.	
White Vinegar	¼ cup	
Butter	1 tbsp.	

Directions

1. Start by boiling the beets until they are tender. Let the beets cool. Once cool, peel and slice the beets into rounds or cut into cubes.
2. Take a small or medium frying pan and mix the salt, sugar, vinegar, and potato starch.
3. Bring it to a boil. Now, reduce the heat and mix in the butter.
4. Finally, pour the sauce over the beets.
5. Either serve immediately or put in the fridge for later.

Nutritional content per serving

Nutrition	Amount per serving
Calories	47.8
Sodium	149.3 milligrams
Protein	0.4 grams
Cholesterol	3.1 milligrams

Potassium	83.9 milligrams
Total Fat	1.2 grams
Carbohydrates	9.5 grams
Saturated Fat	0.7 grams
Fiber	0.5 grams

SWEET POTATO PIE WITHOUT CRUST

Yield	16 servings
Serving size	1 slice

Ingredient	Quantity	Form
Sweet Potatoes	2 cups	Skinless, cooked and mashed
Sugar	1 cup	
Milk	1 cup	Evaporated
Eggs	3	
Butter	2 ½ tbsps.	
Vanilla	1 tsp.	Extract
Cinnamon	1 tsp.	Ground
Nutmeg	A dash	Powder
Cloves	A pinch	Ground
Flour	2 tbsps.	
Salt	1 tsp.	

Directions

1. Start by preheating the oven to 350° F.
2. Next step is to mash the sweet potatoes.
3. Take a bowl and combine all the ingredients and mix well.
4. Once the mixture is ready, pour it into the greased pie tins.
5. Bake at 350 degrees for about 25 to 30 minutes.
6. Allow to cool and serve.

Nutritional content per serving

Nutrition	Amount per serving
Calories	101.3
Sodium	196.6 milligrams
Protein	3.1 grams
Cholesterol	51.3 milligrams
Potassium	132.7 milligrams
Total Fat	3.1 grams
Carbohydrates	15.5 grams
Saturated Fat	1.6 grams
Fiber	0.9 grams

CHEESY CAULIFLOWER MASH

Yield	6 servings
Serving size	½ cup

Ingredient	Quantity	Form
Cauliflower	1 head	Only tips of cauliflower
Butter	2 tbsps.	
Black Pepper	1 tsp.	
Cheddar Cheese	½ cup	Fat free

Directions

1. Start by boiling the cauliflower until its tender.
2. Next step is to drain the cauliflower and add the shredded cheese and butter while the cauliflower is still hot.
3. Finally, add black pepper and mix until you get the desired consistency.

Nutritional content per serving

Nutrition	Amount per serving
Calories	61.3
Sodium	103.3 milligrams
Protein	4.9 grams
Cholesterol	0.0 milligrams
Potassium	135.1 milligrams
Total Fat	0.1 grams
Carbohydrates	4.4 grams
Saturated Fat	0.0 grams
Fiber	1.1 grams

CAULIFLOWER MEATLESS MEATBALLS
(SNACK)

Yield   24 servings
Serving size   1 piece

Ingredient	Quantity	Form
Cauliflower	2 ½ cups	Only tips of cauliflower. Cooked and cut into 1 inch pieces
Eggs	2	Large and fresh
Vegetable Oil	1 tbsp.	
Garlic Powder	½ tsp.	Powder form
Parsley	½ cup	Dry
Parmesan Cheese	½ cup	Grated
Bread Crumbs	½ cup	Plain and dry

Directions

1. Cook the cauliflower until its tender.
2. Now drain as much water off as you can from the cauliflower.
3. Take a bowl and mix all the ingredients together.
4. Form the balls with the help of a tablespoon.
5. Finally, bake at 350 for about 45 minutes until the cauliflower balls are firm and slightly browned.
6. Serve as an appetizer with sauce.

Nutritional content per serving

Nutrition	Amount per serving
Calories	30.9
Sodium	50.1 milligrams
Protein	1.7 grams
Cholesterol	18.8 milligrams
Potassium	39.2 milligrams
Total Fat	1.6 grams
Carbohydrates	2.6 grams
Saturated Fat	0.5 grams
Fiber	0.5 grams

OVEN BAKED SWEET BUTTERNUT SQUASH

Yield   4 servings
Serving size   ½ cup

Ingredient	Quantity	Form
Butternut Squash	1	Medium
Margarine	2 tsp.	Soft
Brown Sugar	1 cup	Unpacked

Directions

1. Start by chopping the stalk off and flower end. Now, chop it in half and lengthwise. Take a spoon and also remove the seeds.
2. Now brush the cut squash with margarine (about 1 tsp. per side).
3. Now, sprinkle the brown sugar and dump the rest into the two holes (about 1/2 cup per side)
4. Finally, bake on the baking tray at 180 degree centigrade for about 30 minutes or until the squash is soft.

    If you notice that the squash starts to brown too much before it is actually cooked, lightly cover it with a foil.

Nutritional content per serving

Nutrition	Amount per serving
Calories	243.1
Sodium	579.5 milligrams
Protein	2.0 grams
Cholesterol	0.0 milligrams

Potassium	765.3 milligrams
Total Fat	2.1 grams
Carbohydrates	58.9 grams
Saturated Fat	0.3 grams
Fiber	0 grams

OVEN BAKED BUTTERNUT SQUASH VERSION 2

Yield   4 servings
Serving size   1 to ½ cups cooked

Ingredient	Quantity	Form
Butternut Squash	1	Medium
Butter Sprays	1-2 per cube	
Salt	As per taste	
Pepper	As per taste	Ground

Directions

1. Start by chopping the stalk off and flower end. Now, chop it in cubes. Take a spoon and also remove the seeds.
2. Place the squash cubes in a 13x9 baking dish and pour in 1/4 inch of water.
3. Finally, cover and bake at 350°F for about 45 minutes or until the squash is tender.

Nutritional content per serving

Nutrition	Amount per serving
Calories	123.0
Sodium	768.0 milligrams
Protein	2.8 grams
Cholesterol	0.0 milligrams
Potassium	873.3 milligrams
Total Fat	0.3 grams
Carbohydrates	32.3 grams
Saturated Fat	0.1 grams

| Fiber | 0 grams |

TURNIP & SQUASH MASH

Yield   4 servings
Serving size 1 cup

Ingredient	Quantity	Form
Turnip	1	Skinless. Cut into same pieces
Butternut Squash	1	Skinless. Cut into same pieces
Natural Buttery Spread	2 tbsp.	Soy garden

Directions

1. Start by chopping the turnip and other root vegetables into the same size pieces.
2. Now, place chopped turnip and root vegetables together in steamer and steam on high heat until they are soft and ready to mash.
3. Once steamed, remove the peel off the vegetables.
4. Finally, drain and return to the pan and mash together with buttery spread.

Nutritional content per serving

Nutrition	Amount per serving
Calories	124.3
Sodium	459.7 milligrams
Protein	1.8 grams
Cholesterol	0.0 milligrams

Potassium	524.0 milligrams
Total Fat	5.7 grams
Carbohydrates	19.1 grams
Saturated Fat	1.8 grams
Fiber	0.8 grams

Chapter 7

Recipes: Beverages

INSTANT RUSSIAN TEA

Yield	5 ½ cups dry powder mix and 88 servings
Serving size	1 tablespoon

Ingredient	Quantity	Form
Tang®	2 cups	
Sugar	½ cup	
Lemonade Mix	1 (2 quart size)	Dry
Instant Tea	1 cup	
Cloves	1 tsp.	
Cinnamon	1 tsp.	Ground

Directions

1. Start by combining all the ingredients.
2. Store the combined ingredients in a covered container.
3. To prepare: add one tablespoon of the mix to about 8-ounces of hot water.
4. Serve hot.

Nutritional content per serving

Nutrition	Amount per serving
Calories	54
Trans Fat	0 grams
Sodium	0 milligrams
Protein	0 grams
Cholesterol	0 milligrams
Potassium	25 milligrams

Total Fat	0 grams
Carbohydrates	13 grams
Phosphorus	17 milligrams
Saturated Fat	0 grams
Fiber	0 grams
Calcium	35 milligrams

HAWAIIAN PUNCH

Yield	8 servings / ½ gallon
Serving size	1 cup or 8-ounces

Ingredient	Quantity	Form
Hawaiian Punch®	1, 48-ounce	Can
Ginger Ale	1, 32-ounce	Bottle

Directions

1. Combine all the ingredients and pour over the ice.
2. Garnish with lime slices or lemon.

Nutritional content per serving

Nutrition	Amount per serving
Calories	103
Trans Fat	0 grams
Sodium	63 milligrams
Protein	1 gram
Cholesterol	0 milligrams
Potassium	47 milligrams
Total Fat	0 grams
Carbohydrates	26 grams
Phosphorus	5 milligrams
Saturated Fat	0 grams
Fiber	0 grams
Calcium	15 milligrams

SPICED UP APPLE JUICE

Yield	8 servings
Serving size	½ cup

Ingredient	Quantity	Form
Nutmeg	½ tsp.	Ground
Cloves	12	Whole
Cinnamon Sticks	4	Broken
Allspice	¼ tsp.	Ground
Apple	1 quart	Unsweetened

Directions

1. Take a saucepan and place all the ingredients in it.
2. Now, slowly bring it to a boil and let it simmer for about 20 minutes.
3. To serve: strain the mix and serve in cups.

Nutritional content per serving

Nutrition	Amount per serving
Calories	63
Trans Fat	0 grams
Sodium	6 milligrams
Protein	1 grams
Cholesterol	0 milligrams
Potassium	132 milligrams
Total Fat	1 grams
Carbohydrates	15 grams
Phosphorus	10 milligrams

Saturated Fat	0 grams
Fiber	1 gram
Calcium	18 milligrams

HERBAL ICED TEA WITH MINT

Yield	8 servings
Serving size	1 cup

Ingredient	Quantity	Form
Herbal Tea	4-5 bags	Fruit flavoured
Boiling Water	4 cups	
Sugar	8 tsps.	
Lemon Juice	1/8 cup	Fresh
Mint	several sprigs	Fresh
Cold Water	5-6 cups	

Directions

1. Take a tea pot and place the tea bags, mint and sugar in it.
2. Now, pour the boiling water and allow steeping for about 15 minutes.
3. Pour it into a pitcher with enough cold water without diluting the concoction too much.
4. Serve.

Nutritional content per serving

Nutrition	Amount per serving
Calories	18.1
Sodium	1.3 milligrams
Protein	0.0 grams
Cholesterol	0.0 milligrams
Potassium	20.1 milligrams
Total Fat	0.0 grams

Carbohydrates	4.9 grams
Saturated Fat	0.0 grams
Fiber	0 grams

MINT LIMEADE

Yield	6 servings
Serving size	1 cup

Ingredient	Quantity	Form
Lime Juice	1 ½ cups	Freshly squeezed
Splenda	1 ½ cups	
Mint Leaves	6	Wooly
Lime Zest	1	
Cold Water	4 cups	

Directions

1. Take a blender and add Splenda, lime juice, mint, zest, and cold water.
2. Also put in a few cubes of ice. Now, blend.
3. Strain and serve cold.

Nutritional content per serving

Nutrition	Amount per serving
Calories	39.4
Sodium	1.2 milligrams
Protein	0.3 grams
Cholesterol	0.0 milligrams
Potassium	72.0 milligrams
Total Fat	0.0 grams
Carbohydrates	5.2 grams
Saturated Fat	0.0 grams
Fiber	0.2 grams

GINGER ICED TEA WITH MINT

Yield	8 servings
Serving size	1 cup

Ingredient	Quantity	Form
Tea Leaves	1 ½ tbsp.	Loose
Ginger	4 slices	Peeled
Lime	1	Sliced
Mint	Few sprigs	Fresh
Boiling Water	1 litre	
Sugar	As desired	
Ice Cubes		
Mint	Extra sprigs	

Directions

1. Take a jug and place the lime, ginger, mint and tea into a jug.
2. Now, pour the boiling water. Let it steep for about 5 minutes.
3. Next step is to strain the mixture into a clean jug and add sugar as per taste. Set it aside and let cool.
4. Serve.

Nutritional content per serving

Nutrition	Amount per serving
Calories	31.2
Sodium	18.1 milligrams
Protein	0.1 grams
Cholesterol	0.0 milligrams
Potassium	36.7 milligrams

Total Fat	0.0 grams
Carbohydrates	8.1 grams
Saturated Fat	0.0 grams
Fiber	0.3 grams

This Page Has Been Left Blank Intentionally.

Chapter 8

Recipes: Desserts

HOMEMADE RIBBON CAKES/COOKIES

Yield	84 cookies
Serving size	2 cookies

Ingredient	Quantity	Form
All-Purpose Flour	3 cups	Unsifted
Sugar	1 cup	
Baking Powder	1 tsp.	
Butter	1 cup	Softened
Eggs	2	
Egg White	1	
Vanilla	½ tsp.	Extract
Plain Jam	1 cup	Seedless. Plum or apricot jam
Sugar	2 tbsp.	

Directions

1. Start by preheating the oven to 375°F.
2. Take a large bowl and combine the flour, sugar, and baking powder.
3. Now, blend in the butter with finger tips until mixture resembles the cornmeal.
4. Now, add the egg whites, eggs and vanilla. Let's now work it into stiff dough.
5. Next step is to divide the dough into two balls, one ball twice the size of the other ball. Take a heavily floured board (about ¼ to ½ cup flour) and roll out the larger ball to 1/8 inches thickness.
6. Now, place the rolled dough in a cookie pan (11" x 15 ½"), smoothing out to edges and patching corners. Now, spread the jelly over the top.

7. Roll out the remaining dough to 1/8 inches thickness and cut into ½ inches wide strips; place the strips diagonally across the jelly, ½ inches apart. Sprinkle sugar over the top and Place in the oven.

8. When the edges start to brown (this will take about 20 minutes), take the pan from the oven, cut of and remove about a 3 inches strip all around the edges. Return the pan to the oven, remove after 10 minutes.

9. Cut into 1" x 2" rectangles. Makes 7 dozen cookies.

Nutritional content per serving

Nutrition	Amount per serving
Calories	106
Trans Fat	1 gram
Sodium	65 milligrams
Protein	1 gram
Cholesterol	14 milligrams
Potassium	17 milligrams
Total Fat	5 gram
Carbohydrates	15 grams
Phosphorus	27 milligrams
Saturated Fat	1 gram
Fiber	0 grams
Calcium	11 milligrams

EGGS CUSTARD

Yield	4 servings
Serving size	½ cup

Ingredient	Quantity	Form
Eggs	2	Medium
Milk	¼ cup	2%
Sugar	3 tbsps.	
Vanilla	1 tsp.	Extract
Nutmeg	1 tsp.	Ground

Directions

1. Start by preheating the oven to 325°F.
2. In an electric mixer, combine all the ingredients, and beat for about one minute until the mixture is thoroughly mixed.
3. Now, pour the mixture into the muffin pans or custard cups.
4. Sprinkle the nutmeg on top.
5. Finally, bake for about 20 to 30 minutes or until a knife inserted into the center of the custard comes out absolutely clean.

Nutritional content per serving

Nutrition	Amount per serving
Calories	70
Trans Fat	0 grams
Sodium	34 milligrams
Protein	3 grams
Cholesterol	91 milligrams

Potassium	30 milligrams
Total Fat	3 grams
Carbohydrates	9 grams
Phosphorus	42 milligrams
Saturated Fat	1 gram
Fiber	0 gram
Calcium	12 milligrams

LEMONY COOKIES

Yield	5 dozen
Serving size	2 cookies

Ingredient	Quantity	Form
Butter	1 cup	Unsalted
Sugar	1 cup	Granulated
Egg	1	
Lemon Extract	1 ½ tsp.	
All-Purpose Flour	1 ½ cup	Sifted

Directions

1. Start by preheating the oven to 375°F.
2. Next step is to cream the butter with sugar.
3. Now, add the egg, lemon extract and beat until it is light and fluffy.
4. Now, add the flour and mix until it is smooth.
5. It's now time to drop the batter by level tablespoon onto the ungreased cookie sheet. Maintain a distance between the cookies of at least 2".
6. Finally, bake the cookies for about 10 minutes or until the cookies brown around the edges.
7. Once done, cool for a minute and remove the cookies from the cookie sheet.

Nutritional content per serving

Nutrition	Amount per serving
Calories	115
Trans Fat	0 grams
Sodium	12 milligrams
Protein	2 gram
Cholesterol	76 milligrams
Potassium	20 milligrams
Total Fat	6 grams
Carbohydrates	12 grams
Phosphorus	23 milligrams
Saturated Fat	1 gram
Fiber	0 grams
Calcium	7 milligrams

GUMDROPS COOKIES

Yield	50 cookies
Serving size	2 cookies

Ingredient	Quantity	Form
Margarine	½ cup	Unsalted and softened
Brown Sugar	1 cup	Packed
Egg	1	Medium
Milk	¼ cup	
Vanilla	1 tsp.	Extract
All-Purpose Flour	1 ¾ cups	Sifted
Baking Powder	1 tsp.	
Gumdrops	15	Large and chopped

Directions

1. Start by preheating the oven to 400°F.
2. Next step is to cream the butter, egg and sugar thoroughly.
3. Now, stir in the vanilla and milk.
4. Take another bowl and mix the flour with baking powder. Once mixed, add flour and baking powder mix to the above ingredients.
5. Now, add and mix in the gumdrops and chill the dough for at least 1 hour.
6. Now, drop the dough by tablespoonful onto the greased cookie sheet.
7. Finally, bake for about 8 to 10 minutes or until the cookies are golden brown.

Nutritional content per serving

Nutrition	Amount per serving
Calories	104
Trans Fat	0 grams
Sodium	9 milligrams
Protein	1 gram
Cholesterol	7 milligrams
Potassium	29 milligrams
Total Fat	1 gram
Carbohydrates	22 grams
Phosphorus	16 milligrams
Saturated Fat	0 grams
Fiber	0 grams
Calcium	13 milligrams

VANILLA ALMOND COOKIES

Yield	75 cookies
Serving size	2 cookies

Ingredient	Quantity	Form
All-Purpose Flour	5 cups	
Butter	2 cups	
Sugar	1 cup and 2 tbsps.	
Eggs	2	
Almond Extract	1 tsp.	
Vanilla	2 tsps.	Extract

Directions

1. Start by preheating the oven to 400°F.
2. Next step is to combine the flour, sugar and butter.
3. Now, add eggs, vanilla extract, almond extract and mix with a hand mixer on low speed or spoon.
4. Now, drop the cookies onto the ungreased baking sheet. You can also use a cookie gun to drop the batter.
5. Finally, bake for about 5 to 8 minutes.
6. Cool before serve.

Nutritional content per serving

Nutrition	Amount per serving
Calories	172
Trans Fat	0 grams
Sodium	56 milligrams

Protein	2 grams
Cholesterol	13 milligrams
Potassium	29 milligrams
Total Fat	7 grams
Carbohydrates	26 grams
Phosphorus	22 milligrams
Saturated Fat	4 grams
Fiber	0 grams
Calcium	8 milligrams

HOMEMADE CREAM CHEESE COOKIES

Yield	7 dozen cookies
Serving size	1 cookie

Ingredient	Quantity	Form
Margarine	1 cup	Softened
Cream Cheese	1, 3-ounce package	Softened
Sugar	1 cup	
Egg Yolk	1	
All-Purpose Flour	2 ½ cups	
Vanilla	1 tsp.	Extract

Directions

1. Start by preheating the oven to 325°F.
2. Next step is to cream the cream cheese and butter. While creaming, slowly add sugar. Keep beating it until fluffy.
3. Now, beat in an egg yolk. Then add the flour and vanilla. Mix everything well.
4. Chill the dough for at least 1 hour.
5. Once chilled, shape the dough into 1 inch balls and place them on the greased cookie sheets.
6. Bake for about 12 to 15 minutes.

Nutritional content per serving

Nutrition	Amount per serving
Calories	80
Trans Fat	0 grams

Sodium	31 milligrams
Protein	0.5 gram
Cholesterol	13 milligrams
Potassium	15 milligrams
Total Fat	4 grams
Carbohydrates	11 grams
Phosphorus	14 milligrams
Saturated Fat	2 grams
Fiber	0 grams
Calcium	6 milligrams

THE POUND CAKE

Yield	24 servings
Serving size	1 slice

Ingredient	Quantity	Form
Margarine	2 cups	Softened
Sugar	4 cups	Powdered
Lemon Rind	2 tbsps.	Grated
Lemon Extract	1 tsp.	
Eggs	6	
All-Purpose Flour	3 ½ cups	Sifted

Directions

1. Start by preheating the oven to 350°F.
2. In an electric mixer, cream the butter for about 3 minutes on medium speed, or until it is light and fluffy.
3. Then gradually add the sugar, lemon rind and cream the mixture thoroughly.
4. Now, add the eggs and lemon extract, one at a time. Mix well after each addition.
5. Gradually add the flour and mix well.
6. Now, pour the mix into the greased and floured 10 inches Bundt pan or tube pan.
7. Now, bake for about 1 hour and 20 minutes or until a wooden pick inserted in center of pound cake comes out absolutely clean.
8. Remove the cake from the pan.
9. Cool and serve.

Nutritional content per serving

Nutrition	Amount per serving
Calories	279
Trans Fat	0 grams
Sodium	127 milligrams
Protein	10 grams
Cholesterol	267 milligrams
Potassium	108 milligrams
Total Fat	11 grams
Carbohydrates	34 grams
Phosphorus	139 milligrams
Saturated Fat	5 grams
Fiber	0 grams
Calcium	40 milligram

HOMEMADE CREAM CHEESE POUND CAKE

Yield	40 cupcakes
Serving size	1 cupcake

Ingredient for Cake	Quantity	Form
Butter	3 sticks	
cream cheese	8 ounces	Softened
Sugar	3 cups	
Vanilla	1 ½ tsp.	Extract
Eggs	4	Large
egg whites	4	Large
white cake flour	3 cups	sifted

Ingredient for Frosting	Quantity	Form
sugar	2, 16-ounce boxes	Powdered
cream cheese	8 ounces	
margarine	½ cup	

Directions

1. Start by preheating the oven to 325°F.
2. Next step is to cream the cream cheese, margarine and sugar until light and fluffy.
3. Then add vanilla extract and beat well.
4. Now, add the eggs, one at a time, and egg whites two at a time, beating well after each addition.
5. Now, stir in the flour.
6. Now, spoon the mixture into a greased and floured muffin pan.

7.   Bake it for about 1 and half hour.
8.   Now, mix the frosting and place it on the cooled cake.

Nutritional content per serving

Nutrition	Amount per serving
Calories	285
Trans Fat	1.7 grams
Sodium	133 milligrams
Protein	3 grams
Cholesterol	6 milligrams
Potassium	29 milligrams
Total Fat	14 grams
Carbohydrates	46 grams
Phosphorus	16 milligrams
Saturated Fat	3 grams
Fiber	0 grams
Calcium	8 milligrams

HOMEMADE WHIPPED CREAME POUND CAKE

Yield   30 slices
Serving size   1 slice

Ingredient for Cake	Quantity	Form
Butter	2 sticks	Softened
Sugar	3 cups	
Eggs	6	
Cake Flour	3 cups	Sifted once before measuring
Whipping Cream	½ pint	
Vanilla	1 tsp.	Extract

Directions

1. Start by preheating the oven to 350°F.
2. Take a tube pan, grease and flour it.
3. Please make sure that all the ingredients of this recipe should be at room temperature.
4. Next step is to cream the margarine and sugar until fluffy.
5. Now, add the eggs, one at a time, beating after each addition.
6. Then, gradually add the flour and whipping cream, blending between each addition.
7. Beat the mixture well for about 30 seconds and then stir in the vanilla flavouring.
8. Finally, pour the batter into the tube pan and bake for about 50 to 60 minutes.

Nutritional content per serving

Nutrition	Amount per serving
Calories	249
Trans Fat	0 grams
Sodium	192 milligrams
Protein	8 grams
Cholesterol	6 milligrams
Potassium	120 milligrams
Total Fat	9 grams
Carbohydrates	35 grams
Phosphorus	24 milligrams
Saturated Fat	2.5 grams
Fiber	0 grams
Calcium	12 milligrams

THE SPICED UP POUND CAKE

Yield	16 slices
Serving size	1 slice

Ingredient for Cake	Quantity	Form
Butter	3 sticks	Softened
Nutmeg	1 ¼ tsp.	Ground
Vanilla	1 tsp.	Extract
Sugar	1 pound	Powdered and Sifted
Eggs	6	
Cake Flour	3 cups	
Sugar	A Little for sprinkle	Powdered

Directions

1. Start by preheating the oven to 325°F.
2. Next step is to take a large bowl and cream the butter until softened.
3. Now, blend in the vanilla extract and nutmeg.
4. Then gradually stir in the powdered sugar.
5. Add the eggs, one at a time, beating well after each addition.
6. Then gradually stir in the flour.
7. Take a 10" x 4" round tube pan, grease only the bottom and flour it lightly. Note: please do not grease the sides of the tube pan.
8. Now, bake for about 1 hour and 20 minutes or until a cake tester inserted in the center comes out absolutely clean.
9. Once done, allow the cake to cool.
10. Once cool, sprinkle with the powdered sugar, cut and serve.

Nutritional content per serving

Nutrition	Amount per serving
Calories	174
Trans Fat	0 grams
Sodium	45 milligrams
Protein	3 grams
Cholesterol	82 milligrams
Potassium	51 milligrams
Total Fat	5 grams
Carbohydrates	33 grams
Phosphorus	25 milligrams
Saturated Fat	2 grams
Fiber	0 grams
Calcium	7 milligrams

FREEZE IT LEMON

Yield	8 squares
Serving size	1 square

Ingredient for Cake	Quantity	Form
Eggs	4	Separated
Sugar	⅔ cup	
Lemon Juice	¼ cup	
Lemon Peel	1 tsp.	Extremely finely grated
Whipping Cream	1 cup	Whipped
Vanilla Wafers	2 cups	Crushed

Directions

1. Start by beating the egg yolks until very thick.
2. Then gradually beat in the sugar. Beat well after each addition.
3. Now, add the lemon peel, lemon juice and blend well.
4. It's time now to cook the mix in a double boiler over hot water stirring constantly until thick.
5. Once cooked, remove it from the heat and allow cooling.
6. Now, beat the egg whites until stiff peaks form.
7. Now, fold in the egg whites into cooled thickened mixture.
8. Now, fold in the whipped cream.
9. Now, take a freezer tray or a 10" x 6" x 1 ½" baking dish and spread 1 and half cups of vanilla wafer crumbs in the bottom.
10. Now, spoon the lemon mixture all over the crumbs.
11. Now, top with the remaining vanilla wafer crumbs.
12. Finally, freeze it for overnight or several hours or until firm.

Nutritional content per serving

Nutrition	Amount per serving
Calories	205
Trans Fat	0 grams
Sodium	97 milligrams
Protein	3 grams
Cholesterol	27 milligrams
Potassium	69 milligrams
Total Fat	7 grams
Carbohydrates	32 grams
Phosphorus	33 milligrams
Saturated Fat	4 grams
Fiber	0 grams
Calcium	22 milligrams

END OF RECIPES

Wrapping Up!

What you eat and drink can drastically ease the symptoms of bowel inflammation or inflammatory bowel disease. Some foods are better for you than others. Cooking and preparing your food from scratch and fresh at home can help you eat healthier and with less fiber.

To help control your fiber intake you will need to avoid high fiber foods, stringy foods and foods with skins and seeds. If you are not sure whether a food is safe to eat, then do not eat it. Prepare the foods you can eat as described in this book and you should be fine. Very fatty foods can be difficult to digest and may cause a lot of discomfort if eaten in the large quantities. Spicy foods may also cause some discomfort and should be avoided.

As low residue diet eliminates lots of fruits and vegetables, it is important that you take enough amount of vitamin C in your diet. In order to vitamin C deficiency, at least have one glass of fruit juice without bits. You can also drink vitamin C enriched fruit drinks or squash, for e.g. orange squash or blackcurrant squash.

At last, I would like to thank you for reading this book and hope that you will create a new healthier you!

RECIPES INDEX

Made in the USA
Lexington, KY
02 December 2016